<u>Forward</u>

C000067234

Why aren't we able to rule ours you'll find out what you're hungry ior. And no diet, no matter how well-planned, will succeed if emotional eating is a factor. You're about to uncover the secret to nutrition mastery, a tried-and-true formula for keeping to any diet you decide is perfect for fulfilling your weight-loss and health-related objectives. know that you're not alone!

"Your emotions are the slaves to your thoughts, and you are the slave to your emotions." Elizabeth Gilbert

"Healthy Eating Healthy Living" isn't a food manual. There are just too many of them. Diets collapse because people cannot stick to them, not because they are ineffective. Learn how to keep on board for every lifestyle, resist binge feeding, and work out what you really desire (hint: it's not food). If you want to avoid emotional eating right now and forever, read all 3 books included in this paperback. Change the hunger for food into a hunger for life!

Are you willing to live a better and happier life than you did in the past? Do you want to start a healthy eating routine in your life?

Then check out these *"Healthy Eating Habits"* that YOU are missing out on!

This book will boost your morale, raise your energy levels, clear your head, and enhance your overall well-being - all so you will begin enjoying a healthier eating lifestyle!

Our lives are full of routine patterns that we follow every day, and these routines form who we are as a result of them. This is why eating well is so crucial in your life. This book will teach you "Healthy Eating Habits" that will fully transform your life. You'll learn what these patterns are and why they're useful to incorporate into your life, as well as a step-by-step Action Plan that teaches you EXACTLY how to put them into practice right away! It's time to drop some weight and appreciate food for what it is: a nutritious and necessary source of energy for your body.

Do you eat to pass the time while you're bored? When you're nervous or stressing out, for example? Is it something you do for the sake of having fun just to stop having to do something else? Or are you the one who needs assistance to overcome this obsessional disorder?

If that's the case, you'll be set free by the facts!

In this book you'll learn how to take off the lies that cause you to overeat and replace them with the reality that will set you free from weight regulation. You'll also learn the What, Why, and solutions of this out-of-reach emotional eating nightmare.

It's not just what you think you had achieved or what you wish you hadn't done. Dunstamac is currently showing you how to reflect on what you Should achieve and how to make things possible. It's a big move further in the right direction. This is the interest of providing you with the fantastically wonderful well-being that you so richly deserve. If so, then this book is for you. It discusses the underlying causes of eating disorders and shows you how to recognize whether or not anyone has an obsession condition and how to cope with it. It's real!

Table of contents

Book 1

Quit Emotional Eating

An Intervention Without the Fluff

Introduction

As a wellness coach, I've done thorough studies on emotional eating and its implications, and I've put together this book with a detailed set of techniques that will hopefully assist you in dealing with your emotional eating habit while also assisting you in being emotionally healthy and independent.

Emotional eating begins at birth as we learn that eating instantly relieves our discomfort (hunger). As humans, we have a propensity to use food to relieve pain. Emotional eating is a pattern in which people use food to help them deal with stressful situations. Several individuals can undergo emotional feeding at any stage in their lives. It - manifests as eating packets of chips when stressed or eating in chocolates after a difficult day at work. However, if emotional eating is done on a daily basis or becomes the primary way a person deals with their emotions, it may have a negative impact on one's health, happiness, and weight. My goal in writing this book is to help you work out how to utilize your inner energies, strengthen your interpersonal relationships, address and resolve stressful stimuli, and show you some emotional eating coping strategies.

To accomplish this goal, I categorized my book into some key parts, each with subsections. In the first segment, I go through some important emotional eating information, followed by subsections on binge eating, emotional and physical hunger, the main causes, and how to cope with them. In the second section, I talk about emotional eating awareness, which includes subsections about why dieting is just a temporary fix for your problems and some solutions that I'll recommend to help you keep hold of your emotional appetite. In the following pages, I'll go through several personal experiences that have helped me regulate emotional eating over time, such as making a journal of your behaviors, maintaining a diet mood diary, and keeping track of your food background. I tie up my book by bringing all of these suggestions together and providing some general guidelines that you might use in a moment of great emotional tension. This coaching book will teach you how to improve your mental health, interact through a multitude of emotional aspects with ease, and cope with feelings effectively without developing emotional eating habits.

Getting on the down-low

By taking a minute to assess your mood, you can begin to reclaim your strength. I've mentioned some key information about emotional eating that you should be aware of. Disturb yourself by finding the answers:

1. What is the concept of binge eating?

BED is characterized by repeated episodes of heavy intake of unusually large amounts of food over a short period of time. These episodes are followed by feelings of guilt, humiliation, and emotional distress. The causes of BED are not well known. Like other eating disorders, it is linked to a variety of environmental, socioeconomic, social, and psychological threats. Overeating compulsively refers to consuming more than is needed. Binge eating disorder is characterized by repeated bouts of compulsive eating that occur even though the person is not hungry. Rapid eating, covert eating, and feeling bad during a binge are also symptoms of bingeing. In the United States, Vyvanse is the only drug licensed to treat binge eating disorder.

1.1. How would it affect you?

BED is related to an increased risk of weight gain and obesity, as well as underlying ailments including diabetes and heart failure. Sleep disturbances, chronic fatigue, mental well-being issues, and a lower standard of living are also potential health risks.

1.2. Difference between Emotional eating and Binge eating

Following are the differences between emotional eating and binge eating.

- Emotional eating is when a person consumes high-carbohydrate, high-calorie foods of little nutritious benefit in reaction to unpleasant emotions such as stress.

- The main distinction between emotional eating and binge eating is the amount of food eaten.

- Emotional eating, like other emotional disorders, is considered to be the product of a combination of causes rather than a particular source.

- Emotional eating, commonly known as panic eating, can show itself in a range of ways.

- Wellness providers check for physical and behavioral health problems when evaluating emotional eating.

- Combating Emotional eating means educating the person on healthy ways to perceive food and build improved eating behaviors (such as conscientious eating), identifying their causes for this behavior, and developing other more appropriate ways to avoid and reduce stress.

- If left unchecked, emotional overeating will contribute to obesity, weight loss issues, and even food abuse.

- Emotional eating can be avoided by reducing depression, eating for nourishment rather than to fix issues, and using constructive approaches to deal with emotions.

1.3. BED is synonymous with bulimia

Fact: Bulimia and BED seem to be identical on the surface. People with the disorders eat excessively and feel anxious, embarrassed, guilty, and out of reach as a consequence of their actions. However, there is one significant distinction between the two scenarios: Bulimia sufferers tend to rid themselves of unnecessary calories by crying, taking laxatives or diuretics (water pills), or over-exercising during a binge.

1.4. What are some of the more popular facts of emotional eating?

There will be certain physical and mental causes for emotional eating. Emotional eating may be triggered by tension or other strong emotions. Coping strategies may assist anyone who is attempting to alleviate more severe symptoms. Just by looking at someone, you can't say whether they have BED. Binge eaters come in a variety of shapes and sizes. What gives that this is possible? Remember that the volume of food and calories are eaten during a "binge" varies from person to person, as does the pace at which calories are burned. Despite this, many individuals with the condition fail to keep a good weight. Obesity is considered to cause around two-thirds of those with the condition.

Other eating disorders, on the other hand, mostly involve women. BED affects both men and women. BED is five times more common in men than any other eating condition. Even if the disorder is related to depressive feelings and increased tension, it's important to note that it's not the same as regular overeating, such as finishing a package of cookies following a split. People with the condition, on the other side, feel tempted to gorge on a daily basis and are unable to regulate their actions.

2. Emotional Hunger vs Physical Hunger

Can you get hungry right away while you're down? Emotional appetite is popular, but it is not the same as physical hunger.

2.1. What is Physical Hunger?

Physical hunger is when the body exhibits hunger signs. And you stop eating when you're uncomfortably whole. Stomach grumbling, feeling weekly or fatigued, hypoglycemia, and feeling lightheaded are all common physical hunger symptoms.

2.2. Stress's physical effect: Increased Food Cravings

Stress is a mental disorder that affects a person's eating and sleeping habits, as well as how they feel about themselves and how they think about problems. Significant depression, dysthymia, and bipolar disorder are the three main forms of depression (also called manic-depressive disease).

There are many physical reasons why a person can overeat as a result of stress and intense emotions:

- **High cortisol levels:** Tension induces the appetite to reduce in order for the body to cope with the crisis. If the stress does not subside, the hormone cortisol is released. Cortisol increases appetite, which may contribute to overeating.

- **Cravings:** Stress-induced rises in cortisol levels can exacerbate food cravings for sweets or unhealthy food. Increased appetite hormones are often linked to fatigue which may contribute to fast food abuse.

- **Gender:** Several studies show that females are more likely than males to use food to deal with stress, while men are far more likely to smoke or drink alcohol.

2.3. What is emotional eating?

Instead of satisfying the needs of the body, emotional hunger is all about eliminating depressive emotions by eating sugary snacks or other calming foods. Comfort foods are usually heavy in sugar and carbohydrates. Anything from work stress to financial issues may be at the center of emotional eating.

2.4. Does emotional eating occur suddenly or gradually?

Emotional deprivation seems to occur suddenly and without warning, and it appears to be immediate. Physical starvation is therefore not as sudden or surprising as it is when a person hasn't eaten for a long time.

2.5. Do you have an addiction to a particular food?

Physical hunger is usually associated with junk food cravings or something unhealthy. Someone who is genuinely starving will still eat something, but anyone who is mentally stressed would want something unusual, such as fries or pizza.

2.6. Is there such a thing as mindless food consumption?

When people consume without paying attention to what they're drinking or eating, it's known as mindless eating.

One example is eating a whole bowl of ice cream while watching TV, despite not planning to eat too much. When it comes to emotional eating, this is a normal phenomenon, as opposed to consuming out of hunger.

2.7. Is hunger perceived in the head or in the stomach?

The stomach may not be the cause of emotional hunger, such as a rumbling and growling stomach. Emotional hunger tends to begin when a person demonstrates an urge or a need for something important to eat.

2.8. Are there any feelings of regret or shame during emotional eating?

By giving in to temptation or eating due to stress, it may trigger feelings of regret, remorse, or guilt. These responses tend to be linked to emotional hunger. Physical hunger, on the other hand, supplies the body with the nutrients or calories it needs to function and is not associated with negative feelings.

3. Emotional Triggers

On any given day, you are likely to encounter a spectrum of emotions, including excitement, unease, frustration, enjoyment, and dissatisfaction. These rules often extend to real-life situations, such as meeting with your boss, talking with a pal about current affairs, or seeing your partner.

The following are examples of situations that can elicit strong emotions

- Betrayed trust
- Inequitable treatment
- Standards that were not fulfilled
- A sense of helplessness or a shortage of supervision
- Left out or forgotten
- Critique or allegation
- Uncomfortable or unneeded thoughts
- The feeling of being surrounded or excessively wanted
- Confusion
- Loss of liberty
- Being turned down

The way you respond to such events can change your emotional status and the circumstances of the situation.

3.1. How to Recognize Yours

Emotional triggers are present in almost all, but they vary in appearance from individual to person. They can include memories of negative past encounters, unpleasant topics, other people's remarks or behavior, or your own behaviors.

Notes:

Awareness

And how would we change anything if we aren't aware of it? As a fitness instructor, I'll share few tips about how to become more mindful of your food patterns and how they affect your mood.

Here are few suggestions for you to remember.

1. The Food History

When you're depressed, do you find yourself reaching for snacks? It's normal for people to look to food for warmth. That is a characteristic of emotional eating. On the other side, physical hunger occurs as the body sends you signals that you are actually starving. Worse, we don't often switch to food to satisfy our thirst. We gorge on such items even too often to alleviate discomfort or other messes. Find out which food cravings will throw your diet off. Food cravings are harmful to the waistline, whether they are creamy or crunchy, sweet or salty. For your health's sake, learn to make healthier dietary decisions.

Keep a journal of all that comes to mind, as well as a record of your emotional past.

Question	Your Response

What was it like at your house during mealtime?

Before going to classes, what did you have for breakfast?

_____

Is it true that the whole family ate dinner together?

_____

What was it like for you?

_____

Were you ever complimented for your eating skills?

_____

Have you ever been chastised for being a picky eater?

_____

Were you hungry all of the time or just occasionally?

_____

What are large family get-together's, such as holidays?

_____

What are the plans for the holidays?

_____

Did you seek solace from food?

_____

When did it all begin?

_____

When you were overweight?

_____

When did they first start?

_____

If you have some particular things that you crave?

_____

When did this begin?

_____

What did your caregivers think about your dietary habits?

_____

What were the messages you sent yourself about your eating habits?

_____

Have you developed a binge eating problem?

_____

If so, when do you think that would happen?

_____

Do you ever feel out of balance when it comes to food?

_____

If that's the case, where did it start?

_____

Has diet been a healthy haven for you?

_____

When did it begin?

_____

Do you have any children?

_____

What was your reaction to them in terms of food?

_____

How did the kids handle mealtime?

Are you now doing the "See Food" diet: see it, eat it!

Are you bombarded with health and food commercials?

If that's the case, which one is it?

Will you refrain from consuming such foods (junk food)?

As long as it is not in focus?

If you have a habit of paying for your meals?

Did you go on a diet? Effectively or unsuccessfully?

2. The Food-Mood Diary

One of the first steps to increase consciousness is to pay close attention to what you consume. If you're reading this after you've already consumed a meal or two, you should begin right now. What did you have for dinner? Assess the day to the highest possible norm. When are you going to do it? Are you aware of any stimulating occurrences or emotions when you eat? If you continue to do this, you may become more conscious of the triggering experiences and emotions that will cause you to feed.

("Fill in the sheet any time you consume anything in the next thirty days (yes, even one nibble of something counts)").

Time/ Date	Food	Event	Mood

Quit Emotional Eating

3. Your Journal

Keeping a journal will help you deal with mental eating disorders in a therapeutic manner. I maintained a journal of my private thoughts and emotions for several years. I always began a page by writing, "I don't know what to write about today." My pen was gliding over the paper in a few minutes, leaving a trail of words in its path. I let the words flow freely on the paper, feeling everything that was bubbling up inside of me. I didn't worry about spelling or punctuation; I just let my hand keep writing until it was exhausted. The time was spent, but it was spent more happily. Writing has been extremely therapeutic for me. For a couple of months, keep a diet journal. Create a note of what you consume and why you eat everything. It will assist you in defining your patterns. You may find, for example, that you crave a sweet snack to help you through the mid-afternoon energy low. It's important to keep track of how you felt when you wanted to eat, particularly if you ate when you weren't hungry. Were you exhausted? Are you feeling tense?

Instead of eating your emotions, start writing them down in a journal. You can write whatever you want and keep writing until you have a clear picture of yourself. When you write for at least 15 minutes every day, you'll soon discover the magic of keeping a journal!

Your journal

4. Diets are a self-contained, temporary cure

The irony is that these interventions are ineffective because the deeper issues are not addressed. Diets, for example, fail because they focus solely on the level of shallow behavior. People are led to believe that if they just lose weight, their lives will improve, their depression will subside, and that once the diet is over, they will magically become relaxed around food. If you're reading this, you've probably already admitted to yourself that dieting only makes things worse. Abstinence from food addiction entails ceasing to engage in the behaviors associated with your eating disorder, such as binge eating, obsessing over food, limiting, and all other behaviors associated with your specific type of food or eating addict.

5. The Union

Whatever you do, whether it's your dietary patterns, how you drink everything you buy, or how you feel for your body, happens for whatever purpose. It's called the superficial stage because it's not the cause of the problem; although it is a problem, it's just what's closer to the top. The issue isn't one of food. The issues arise from the way food is consumed. If you never reform your habits, you'll just be able to change them for a short time. To have a better understanding of what motivates you to use food the way you do, dig a little deeper.

Self-Care

1. Breathing slowly

If you're deliriously cheerful or so sad that you can't talk, the force of a deep breath has a lot to say. Slowing things down and paying attention to what's going on won't help the feelings go away fast (and realize, that is not the goal).

- **Take a deep breath in slowly:** The diaphragm, not the lung, takes deep breaths. Visualize your breath slowly rising from deep inside your belly button. Yeah, you've got it. Hold the breath for three counts, and slowly release it.

- **Think of the mantra**: Hearing a mantra, such as "I am calm" or "I am peaceful," maybe calming to certain people.

2. Offer Some Space to Yourself

Taking the time away from intense feelings, in my opinion, can help you ensure that you are listening to them rationally. This chasm could be emotional, such as quitting an upsetting circumstance. However, by occupying yourself, you will also develop self-esteem.

While you don't want to totally suppress or stop feelings, it's not harmful to distract yourself while you're in a better mood to deal with them. Just make sure you're on your way back to them. Healthy distractions are just temporary.

3. Try Some Distractions

Take a hike, enjoy a good show, talk to a loved one, pet the cat for a few minutes, catch as much sleep as possible, create time for friends to chat (and laugh), exercise, spend time with loved ones, and find time for relaxation and hobbies.

If you've figured out what you're doing, you'll be able to approach and learn from those emotions that are more well established.

4. Meditation

If you aren't currently seeing a psychiatrist, that might be one of the better choices for coping with extreme feelings. Meditation will help you develop a deeper view of your emotions and experiences. When meditating, you teach yourself to calm down with those feelings, to notice them without judging yourself or trying to alter or remove them.

It can foster emotional regulation by teaching you to understand all of your feelings, as mentioned above. Meditation helps you to develop your acceptance skills. It also has other benefits, such as assisting you in relaxing and sleeping well.

5. Self-Care Activity

It is important that we have a greater understanding of ourselves! What self-care habits would you love to incorporate into your everyday routine? Any suggestions: Relax in a hot bath with candles or bath salts. Only enjoy a nice time. Pour yourself a cup of coffee and sit back for five minutes. For ten minutes, don't do something until you've had a cup of tea. Make a list right now.

6. Identify Toxic Relationship

When it comes to managing emotional stimuli, you have a lot of leverage. Your answers are not the liability of someone else. They are, moreover, responsible for their behavior, which can lead you to feel upset. So, as a coach, my advice is to recognize those individuals and stay away from them.

7. Supporting Group

"Finding supporting people or forming a social network satisfies our fundamental desire to belong."

Start recognizing the people who can help you. These are the ones who can listen to you without passing judgment and will be there to support you.

First, you have to list down the qualities you are seeking in your support group as following:

1. ---------------------- 6. ----------------------

2. ---------------------- 7. ----------------------

3. ---------------------- 8. ----------------------

4. ---------------------- 9. ----------------------

5. ---------------------- 10. ----------------------

Then list the people who fit these qualities, and list them as follows:

1. --

2. --

3. --

4. --

5. --

Conclusion

Putting all of the above into consideration, the most common causes cited by people are loneliness, schedules, exhaustion, and social pressures. The first phase in overcoming emotional eating is to understand the causes and circumstances that arise in one's life. Holding a food diary or document may help pinpoint periods that someone is overeating due to emotional hunger rather than physical hunger. Anyone may gain insight into their eating patterns by tracking their behavior.

They'd like to brainstorm suggestions about how to fix their proven causes next. Anyone who eats when stressed, for example, might start learning a new book that sounds fascinating or starting a new challenging task. To help themselves deal with their feelings, anyone who consumes due to stress can prefer to meditate, rest, or go for a walk. Anyone who emotionally eats can attempt to call a friend, take their dog for a walk, or schedule an adventure to deal with their "bad feelings" while they are depressed. Try using all of the above techniques to see how the emotional eating preferences shift.

Book 2

Healthy Eating Habits

A Guide to Tweaking and Balancing

the Regular Diet

(Weight Loss, Low Carb, Sugar,

Diet, Metabolism, Cravings)

Introduction

Food provides the nutrition that our bodies need to survive. Food is indeed a matter of history and custom. This may indicate that eating has an emotional aspect. Changing one's eating habits is difficult for many individuals.

You may not be aware that these food behaviors are dangerous because you have been doing them for a long time. Alternatively, your patterns have been so entrenched in your everyday routine that you don't owe them much consideration. We have a good deal of behaviors when it comes to food. Some are positive ("I always eat breakfast"), and others are negative ("I always clean my plate"). Since much of our eating patterns are formed during adolescence, it is never too late to make a shift.

With so many items and weight-loss theories on the market, it's easy to get perplexed. I've added a section on 'diet myths and reality' to help you escape a lot of the misinformation that muddles our minds around dieting and eating well. The details in this book will help to debunk misconceptions about weight loss, diet, and physical activity. Living a healthier lifestyle can become the second standard if we build improved eating habits. Learn how to eat healthily while avoiding unnecessary drama and fluff.

The jumble of good fats versus poor fats, easy meals versus slow-cooked foods, and what-to-eat and what-not-to-eat updates would undoubtedly overwhelm you in your quest to get active and balanced. The decision on whether to eat then becomes a major fight.

When it comes to healthier living, often individuals have the same challenges and concerns. You've already received contradictory reports from a variety of sources, and you now believe you have no idea what good eating entails. Then you start asking yourself a lot of questions.

This book will show you...

1. The significance of a balanced diet

2. Taking care of your eating in the proper manner

3. How to correctly search for nutritious foods

4. When do you take supplements?

5. How to eat healthily without relying on menus or complicated instructions

6. Maintain a safe lifestyle even though you're out and about or on vacation.

7. Ingenious strategies to get the kids to consume nutritious meals

In this book, some bad eating habits are discussed with detailed solutions. In the pages below some healthy foods, habits, and strategies are discussed, these will definitely help you to return to a healthy lifestyle. You'll be motivated to make smarter decisions and live your life to the fullest extent possible.

Chapter 1.   Eating Habits

Eating habits (also known as dietary habits) relate to when and how individuals consume, what foods they eat, and from whom they eat, as well as how they receive, store, use, and dump food. Individuals' eating habits are influenced by a variety of variables including social, cultural, religious, fiscal, environmental, and political factors.

Why and How People Eat?

Humans must eat in order to live. They even eat to show gratitude, to feel a sense of belonging, to follow family traditions, and to achieve self-realization. Someone who is not hungry, for example, may eat a slice of cake baked in his or her honor.

People eat according to etiquette, meal and snack patterns, acceptable foods, food combinations, and portion sizes that they have learned. Acceptable behaviors are referred to as etiquette. For example, some cultures consider it acceptable to lick one's fingers while eating, while others consider it impolite. Depending on whether the meal is formal, informal, or special, etiquette and eating rituals differ (such as a meal on a birthday or religious holiday).

A meal is typically defined as the consumption of two or more foods at a predetermined time in a structured setting. Snacks are small portions of food or beverages consumed in between meals. Three meals (breakfast, lunch, and dinner) per day, with snacks in between, is a common eating pattern. A meal's components vary by culture, but they typically include grains like rice or noodles, meat or a meat substitute like fish, beans, or tofu, and side dishes like vegetables. Various food guides offer advice on what to eat, how much to eat, and how much to drink on a daily basis. Personal preferences, habits, family customs, and social setting, on the other hand, heavily influence what a person consumes.

What do people eat?

There are acceptable and unacceptable foods in every culture, but this is not determined by whether or not something is edible. Alligators, for example, are found in many parts of the world, but many people refuse to eat them. Horses, turtles, and dogs, for example, are eaten (and even considered delicacies) in some cultures but are not acceptable food sources in others. There are also rules about who it is acceptable to eat with. Doctors in a healthy hospital, for example, can eat in different areas from patients or customers.

Getting, Preserving, Consuming, and Tossing Away Food

Food is obtained, preserved, and discarded in a number of forms by humans. Any food is grown, fished, or hunted, while the majority is purchased from supermarkets or specialized stores. People can store small amounts of food and get the majority of what they eat on a daily basis if they have limited access to energy sources. People who live in houses with plenty of room and electricity, on the other hand, buy food in bulk and store it in freezers, refrigerators, and pantries. In any scenario, appropriate disposal facilities are needed to prevent environmental and health issues.

Exposure to Food

There are a plethora of spices and cuisine varieties to choose from. Some tastes or food blends are easy to consider, whereas others must be developed or studied. Sweetness is widely liked, but a palate for salty, savory, spicy, sour, bitter, and hot flavors must be created. The more a human is introduced to food and motivated to consume it, the more likely they are to consider it. If a person's sensitivity to food rises, they become more comfortable with it and less afraid of it, and approval may grow. Some people consume only such foods and flavor blends, while others enjoy experimenting with new foods and tastes.

Chapter 2. Influences on Food Choices

There are numerous factors that influence what food an individual eats. There are cultural, social, religious, technological, environmental, and even political considerations in addition to personal interests.

2.1. Individual Preferences

When it comes to cooking, everybody has their own tastes. Personal interactions such as motivation to consume, introduction to a diet, family customs and traditions, advertisement, and personal beliefs all affect these habits over time. For example, despite the fact that frankfurters are a family tradition, one individual may dislike them.

2.2. Cultural Influences

Appropriate items, food combinations, eating habits, and eating practices are all described by a cultural community. Individuals that follow these rules develop a sense of self-identity and belonging. Subgroups occur within broad ethnic groups that may follow variants of the larger group's eating habits while also being deemed a member of the larger group. An average American meal, for example, consists of a hamburger, French fries, and a beer. In the United States, though, vegetarians consume "veggie-burgers" made from mashed beans, pureed tomatoes, or soy, and dieters may eat a lean turkey burger. There are acceptable cultural substitutions in the United States, but a horsemeat burger will be unethical.

2.3. Social Influences

A social group's members are reliant on one another, share a shared community, and affect one another's attitudes and beliefs. Food habits are influenced by a person's participation in specific peer, career, or neighborhood groups. For example, at a basketball game, a young person might consume some foods with his or her friends and other foods with his or her instructor.

2.4. Religious influences

The number of religious prohibitions varies greatly, from a few to a large number, and from casual to rigid. And would have an effect on a follower's eating habits and attitudes. For example, some items are forbidden in certain sects, such as pork among Jewish and Muslim followers. Under Christianity, Seventh-day Adventists discourage the use of "stimulating" drinks such as beer, which is not prohibited by Catholics.

2.5. Economic Influences

What an individual buys, is influenced by money, beliefs, and customer skills. The cost of a meal, on the other hand, is not a reliable measure of its nutritional value. The cost of food is calculated by a dynamic mixture of its supply, status, and demand.

2.6. Environmental Influences

The climate has an effect on eating patterns due to a combination of ecological and social influences. Foods that are widely available and easy to grow in a particular area often become part of the local cuisine. Many foods that were formerly only accessible during those seasons or in certain areas are now available virtually everywhere, at any time, thanks to new technologies, farming techniques, and transportation methods.

2.7. Political Influences

Food supply and patterns are often affected by political influences. Food policies and trade deals have an effect on what is accessible inside and across nations, as well as on food costs. Consumers' awareness of the food they buy is determined by food labeling rules.

Eating patterns are thus influenced by both external and internal influences, such as politics and morals. These patterns are developed over a person's lifespan and can alter.

Chapter 3.   Diet and Nutrition

3.1.   Bad Eating Habits and How to Break Them

Snacking late at night, emotional eating, and junk-food binges ring a bell? Breaking these typical poor eating patterns will help you lose weight quickly.

Overeating and weight gain were caused by more than just a loss of motivation. It's also the sly poor habit you picked up without even noticing it, like rushing out the door without eating some mornings or munching chips while watching your favorite TV program. The next thing you know, one little poor behavior has added up to a large amount of weight gain. Worst of all, you might not even be aware of what you're doing to your diet.

Here are several fast remedies for some of the more popular dietary and lifestyle patterns that can lead to weight gain.

3.1.1.   The Bad Habit: Mindless Eating

Brian Wansink, Ph.D., a Cornell University food psychologist, found that the bigger the plate or cup you feed on, the more you unconsciously drink. Wansink discovered in a recent survey that moviegoers who were provided extra-large containers of expired popcorn nevertheless consumed 45 percent more than those who ate fresh popcorn from smaller containers containing the same number.

The Solution: Consume food from smaller plates. Try using a salad plate instead of a big dinner plate, and never eat directly from a cup or box.

3.1.2.   The Bad Habit: Eating Late at Night

According to diet folklore, eating late at night is almost never a smart thing if you're trying to lose weight. Despite the fact that many scientists assume this old adage is a fallacy, a recent animal report reinforces the notion that it's not only what you consume, but even what you eat that matters. Mice fed high-fat diets throughout the day (when these nocturnal animals could have been sleeping) gained slightly more weight than mice fed the same diet at night, according to Northwestern University researchers.

The Solution: Is this a diet take-out joint? After dinner, tell yourself that the kitchen is locked for the night and brush your teeth — a freshly washed mouth may make you want to eat less. Wait 10 minutes if you have a craving. If you're ever hungry, take a quick snack such as string cheese or a slice of fruit.

3.1.3.   The Bad Habit: Excessive Snacking

Snacking around the clock, mostly on high-calorie snacks high in empty carbohydrates, is a terrible habit that many people have. It's not just a challenge for adults, according to a new survey from the University of North Carolina: kids are snacking more and more on unhealthy fast food like fatty snacks, soda, and sweets.

According to Jessica Crandall, RD, a spokesperson for the American Dietetic Association, hold only nutritious snacks within scopes, such as hummus, carrots and cucumber sticks, air-popped popcorn, milk, and almonds. Don't have potato chips or treats on your desk or in your pantry that you know you'll eat.

3.1.4. The Bad Habit: Skipping Breakfast

You realize that breakfast is the most important meal of the day, however, you may decide that you don't have time to eat because you have too many other things to do. When you miss meals, your metabolism slows down, according to Crandall, and breakfast offers you the injection of energy you need to get through the day. You'll definitely overeat later if you don't have this power. Over a two-year stretch, Chinese schoolchildren who missed breakfast gained slightly more weight than those who consumed a morning meal, according to a new report.

The Solution: Get nutritious breakfast snacks on hand so you can eat on the go, according to Crandall. If you're short of time, go for simple foods like whole berries, milk, homemade cereal bars, and smoothies.

3.1.5. The Bad Habit: Emotional Eating

You've had a tough day at work, but when you get home, you open the refrigerator and consume something unhealthy — not a smart eating plan. Crandall explains, "You bring food in your mouth as a calming mechanism." A variety of studies show that people's feelings, both good and negative, may encourage them to consume more than they should, which is a common weight-loss roadblock.

The Solution: According to Crandall, is to discover a different stress reliever. "If you're stressed out at college, go for a stroll instead of eating or call a sympathetic buddy when you get home "she proposes "You will let off steam and relieve some of the stress." You can do anything you want as long as it takes you away from the kitchen.

3.1.6. The Bad Habit: Eating too Fast

If you're snacking or enjoying a meal, wolfing down the food doesn't allow your head time to catch up with your stomach. It takes 15 to 20 minutes for your brain to register that you're complete once you've stopped eating. If you consume your meal in less than 10 minutes, you can consume much more than you need. Japanese researchers discovered that consuming very fast was closely linked to becoming overweight in a survey of 3,200 men and women.

The Solution: To eat more slowly, place your fork down between bites, take smaller bites, and chew each bite thoroughly. Additionally, consuming water after the meal can assist you in slowing down and feeling fuller.

3.1.7. The Bad Habit: Not Getting Enough Sleep

Is it possible that not having enough sleep would sabotage the weight-loss efforts? Yes, according to a new study conducted by Tokyo researchers. Men and women who slept five hours or less a night were shown to be more likely to gain weight than someone who slept seven hours or more a night.

The Solution: Establish a daily schedule for yourself, and aim to go to bed and wake up at the same time every day, except on weekends. Keep the space quiet and warm, and stop watching TV or using laptops for at least an hour before heading to bed. If you need more inspiration to go to bed early, keep in mind that the better you sleep, the better the number on the scale would be in the morning.

3.1.8. The Bad Habit: Vegging Out with Video Games

Whether you're watching TV, seated in front of a monitor, or playing video games, you don't just have to think about mindless snacking in front of the television. According to a recent survey, teenagers who spent one-hour playing video games consumed more the remainder of the day, resulting in weight gain. The researchers aren't exactly why boys who play video games consume more, although they believe that sitting in front of a screen all day could have a similar impact on adults, leading to snacking.

The Solution: Take regular breaks from the screen — 45 to 60 minutes, get up, and move around the space or workplace. When the workday or your favorite TV program is done, try to keep track of what you eat so you don't overeat.

3.1.9.   The Bad Habit: Eating Junk Food

You may realize that fast food is bad for your waistline, but the result might be much greater. Several experimental experiments also discovered that high-fat, high-sugar diets are toxic to rats' brains, comparable to cocaine or heroin. Another research discovered that consuming comfort food really makes people feel happy.

The Solution: According to research, excluding your favorite indulgences from your diet would just help you miss them more. The trick to weight reduction success is to figure out what you really desire and only enjoy it in the balance as unique treats rather than every day.

Chapter 4.   Eat well

The trick to a healthier diet is to obtain the appropriate number of calories for your level of activity so that the nutrition you take is balanced with the energy you expend. You can accumulate weight if you eat unhealthily or consume more than the body requires and the nutrition you cannot use is retained as fat. You can lose weight if you eat and drink too little. You can also eat a number of foods to guarantee that you have a well-balanced diet and that the body is having all of the nutrients it needs.

Men can eat roughly 2,500 calories a day (10,500 kilojoules). A woman's daily calorie intake should be about 2,000 calories (8,400 kilojoules). The majority of adults in the United Kingdom consume more calories than they require and can consume fewer calories.

4.1. Useful tips to eat well

These eight useful tips cover the foundations of safe eating and will assist you in making smart decisions.

4.1.1. Eat more high-fiber starchy carbs

Just over a portion of your diet can be made up of starchy carbohydrates. Potatoes, bread, rice, noodles, and cereals are among them. Choose wholewheat spaghetti, brown rice, or potatoes with their skins on for higher fiber or wholegrain types.

They have more fiber than white or processed starchy carbs, but they will keep you feeling fuller much longer. With each main meal, try to provide at least one starchy food. Some people believe starchy foods are fattening, but the carbohydrate they produce contains less than half the calories of a fat gram.

When frying or serving these things, keep an eye on the fats you use because this is what lifts the calorie count – for example, oil on chips, butter on toast, and creamy sauces on pasta.

4.1.2. Consume a variety of fruits and vegetables

Every day, you can consume at least 5 portions of a number of fruits and vegetables. They come in a range of ways, including raw, frozen, bottled, dry, and juiced. Having that 5 A Day is not as complicated as it may seem. Replace your mid-morning snack with a slice of fresh fruit by chopping a banana over your breakfast cereal.

80g is a serving of natural, dried, or frozen fruit and vegetables. 30g of dried fruit (which can be served mainly at mealtimes). A 150ml glass of fruit juice, vegetable juice, or smoothie counts as one serving, just restrict yourself to one glass per day since these beverages are rich in sugar and will damage your teeth.

4.1.3. Increase the seafood consumption, including a part of fatty fish

Fish is high in calcium and includes a variety of vitamins and minerals. Aim to consume at least two servings of fish each week, each of which should be oily.

Omega-3 fats found in oily fish can help to prevent heart disease.

Fish that are high in oil include:

1. Salmon

2. trout

3. herring

4. sardines

5. pilchards

6. mackerel

Fish that aren't oily include:

- haddock

- plaice

- coley

- cod

- tuna

- skate

- hake

Note: New, frozen, and packaged fish are all options, but canned and smoked fish include a lot of salt. While most people can consume more fish, certain varieties of fish have proposed restrictions.

4.1.4. Minimize the amount of saturated fat and sugar in the diet

Saturated fat is an unhealthy kind of fat. You need fat in your diet, but the quantity and form of fat you consume must be carefully monitored. Saturated and unsaturated fats are the two major categories of fat. Over much-saturated fat in your diet will raise your blood cholesterol levels, increasing your risk of heart disease.

Note: Men can consume no more than 30 grams of saturated fat a day on average. Women can eat no more than 20 grams of saturated fat a day on average.

Kids under the age of 11 should consume fewer saturated fat than adults, but children under the age of 5 should not consume a low-fat diet.

Saturated fat can be present in a number of foods, including:

- fatty cuts of meat

- sausages

- butter

- hard cheese

- cream

- cakes

- biscuits

- lard

- pies

Reduce the consumption of saturated fats and replace them with unsaturated fats from things like edible oils and spreads, fatty fish, and avocados. Using a small amount of vegetable or olive oil, or a reduced-fat spread instead of butter, lard, or ghee for a healthy substitute. When eating meat, choose lean cuts and trim away any noticeable fat. Since all forms of fat are rich in calories, they should be consumed in moderation.

4.1.5. Sugar

Eating high-sugar foods and beverages on a daily basis increases the chance of obesity and tooth loss. Sugary foods and beverages are rich in energy (measured in kilojoules or calories) and can lead to weight gain if drunk too often. They may also induce tooth decay if consumed in between meals.

Sugars applied to foods or beverages, as well as sugars contained naturally in butter, syrups, and unsweetened fruit juices and smoothies, are also examples of free sugars. Rather than the sugar present in fruits and milk, this is the kind of sugar you should be avoiding. Free sugars are present in surprising quantities in many foods and beverages.

Free sugars can be present in a variety of foods, including:

- sugary fizzy drinks

- sugary breakfast cereals

- cakes

- biscuits

- pastries and puddings

- sweets and chocolate

- alcoholic drinks

Food labeling may be useful. Use them to determine how much sugar is in foods. Food with more than

22.5g of total sugars per 100g is heavy in sugar, whereas food with less than 5g of total sugars per 100g is poor in sugar. Learn how to reduce the amount of sugar in your diet.

4.1.6. Limit the salt intake to no more than 6 grams a day for adults

Too much salt in your diet will increase your blood pressure. High blood pressure makes you more likely to have heart problems or experience a stroke. You could be consuming too much even though you don't add salt to your diet.

Around three-quarters of the salt, you ingest is already found in items such as breakfast cereals, soups, bread, and sauces before you purchase them.

To help you save from salts, look at product labeling. The presence of more than 1.5g of salt per 100g suggests that the food is salty. Adults and children aged 11 and up can consume no more than 6g (approximately a teaspoonful) of salt a day. Kids under the age of six can have much fewer.

4.1.7. Keep exercising and sustain a healthier weight.

Daily exercise, in addition to eating healthily, can help lower your risk of developing serious health problems. It's also crucial for good fitness and happiness.

Type 2 diabetes, some tumors, cardiac failure, and stroke may also be caused by being overweight or obese. Being underweight will have a detrimental effect on your well-being. Most people need to reduce their calorie intake in order to lose weight.

If you wish to lose weight, strive to eat less and do more. Maintaining a good weight may be as easy as consuming a healthy, nutritious diet. Use the BMI balanced weight calculator to see whether you're at a healthy weight. Begin the NHS weight-loss program, a 12-week plan that incorporates a balanced diet with physical exercise guidance. See underweight adults if you're underweight. If you're nervous about your weight, contact your doctor or a dietitian.

4.1.8. Do not get thirsty

To avoid being dehydrated, you can consume lots of water. The government advises that you consume 6 to 8 glasses of water a day. This is in comparison to the fluid you ingest from your food.

Both non-alcoholic beverages are appropriate, but water, low-fat milk, and low-sugar beverages, such as tea and coffee, are better alternatives. Sugary soft and fizzy beverages are rich in calories, so skip them. They're even detrimental to your dental health. Free sugar is included in still unsweetened fruit juice and smoothies.

Your regular total of beverages including fruit juice, vegetable juice, and smoothies does not reach 150ml, which is around half a bottle. If it's sunny outside or you're running, try to take some water.

4.1.9. Do not skip breakfast

Some people say missing breakfast can help them lose weight. A nutritious breakfast rich in fiber and low in calories, sugar, and salt, on the other hand, will help you get the nutrients you need for good health as part of a regular diet. A delicious and healthier breakfast is whole grain lower-sugar cereal with semi-skimmed milk and fruit slices on top.

Conclusion

This book "Healthy Eating Habits" will assist you in achieving a healthy lifestyle. Often, think of the good behaviors you already have and be aware of them. Learn not to be overly hard on yourself when it comes to your acts. It's quick to get caught up in your bad habits. This will cause you to get stressed and give up on your efforts to improve.

The first meal of the day sets the pace for the rest of the day. A filling, balanced meal can supply the body with the resources it takes to bring you to lunch. If you're not hungry when you wake up, a glass of milk or small fruit and dairy-based smoothie may be a decent choice. We also have exercise and diet aspirations when it comes to our well-being, such as gaining weight, exercising more, eating healthy, or making smart food decisions. It might take months to lose weight. Daily exercise may take years, although eating healthy and making informed dietary decisions are impossible to calculate. We will become frustrated and give up before achieving these objectives. To keep on track, we should break down our fitness objectives into simpler, more achievable measures - steps that are easy to calculate and track weekly or monthly so we can see our success and stay inspired.

If you find yourself resuming an old routine, consider why you did so. Replace that with a fresh habit once more. You are not a loser because you made a mistake. Continue to pursue!

Book 3

Emotional Eating - Myth vs Reality

The What? The Why?

and Solutions of Emotional Eating

Introduction

Emotional eating may be soothing in the short term, but in this book we expose why it's not the healthiest choice in the long run. If you're an emotional eater, you might eat to relieve tension and depression, increase pleasure, and provide warmth. Overeating, on the other side, adds to weight gain, heart failure, asthma, and a slew of other health concerns. Here are some Myths and Realities about emotional eating that should make you rethink how you deal with life's stressors, disappointments, and other feelings.

Overeating isn't uncommon — just think about Thanksgiving, as you stuff yourself silly. Although there's a major gap between occasional overeating and binge eating disorder, which is a psychiatric disease (BED). Binge eating is associated with feelings of depression, shame, and powerlessness. It's not about partying — that's probably one of the many stereotypes about this illness. Here we will discuss the strategies and some coping techniques that will help you to be emotionally independent.

Emotional eating isn't about meeting the body's basic nutritional requirements for energy. It's about saturating the blood with carbohydrates on a regular basis, as a result of a loss of emotional discipline, a profound psychiatric illness that must be bravely confronted and medically monitored.

While diets have existed since Adam and Eve had to reduce their dessert choices, it wasn't until the 1960's that our collective consciousness around weight loss moved into high gear. It expanded to our current degree of fascination within a few decades. We consume more food-related content and have more representations of food in the media and climate than the majority of the world's population. This relentless emphasis on diet and weight will only help to enhance the latent urge to overeat.

It is important that we learn to manage tension in our daily lives. Emotional eating can't be completely eliminated and it's a function of everyday life. We should, however, learn to relieve stress, anxiety using strategies like exercise, mindfulness, yoga, time management, and support programs, giving us more power over our already set eating behaviors and their impacts on our physical and mental well-being.

Chapter 1. Emotional Eating - Causes and Facts

Emotional eating is the urge of sufferers to eat in response to unpleasant or difficult thoughts, particularly though they are not physically hungry. Mental eating, also known as emotional appetite, is characterized by a need for high-calorie or high-carbohydrate items with little nutritional benefit. Comfort snacks, such as ice cream, cakes, chocolate, popcorn, French fries, and pizza, are often craved by emotional eaters. When anxious, about 40% of people eat more, 40% eat less, and 20% eat the same volume. As a result, depression is linked to both weight gain and weight loss.

Although emotional eating may be a sign of atypical depression, often individuals who do not have psychiatric depression or any other mental health disorder partake in this behavior in reaction to fleeting emotions or long-term stress. This is a very normal condition that is critical because it may make it impossible to follow a healthier diet and lead to obesity.

Is It Really That Depression Makes You Fat?

The Stress Hormone Cortisol

Since excess cortisol is secreted at periods of physical or psychological discomfort, and the usual cycle of cortisol secretion (with amounts greatest in the morning and lowest at night) may be disrupted, cortisol has been dubbed the "stress hormone." Cortisol secretion destruction can not only facilitate weight gain, but it may also influence where the weight is stored in the body. According to some research, depression and high cortisol levels affect fat accumulation in the abdomen region rather than the hips. Since abdominal fat deposition is closely connected to the occurrence of cardiovascular disease, including heart attacks and strokes, this fat deposition has been nicknamed "toxic fat."

When it comes to emotional eating and binge eating, what's the difference?

The volume of food eaten is the main distinction between emotional eating and binge eating. Although all include a feeling of difficulty suppressing a food craving, emotional eating can involve consuming small or large amounts of food and maybe the only sign of a mental condition such as obesity, bulimia, or binge eating disorder, or it may be a result of one. Binge eating disorder is a psychiatric condition marked by repeated periods of compulsive overeating in which affected individuals ingest a quantity of food that is far greater than what other people consume in a specific time frame (for example, over two hours) except though they are not hungry. An individual suffering from a binge eating disorder can eat far more quickly than normal, hide the amount they eat out of embarrassment and feel disgusted by their food afterward. The binges must occur on average once a week over three months to apply for this condition.

What are the causes, triggers, and risk factors?

Emotional eating, like other emotional signs, is considered to be the product of a combination of causes rather than a particular source. Girls and women are at a greater risk for eating disorders, according to some studies, and they are often at a higher risk for emotional eating. Another study shows that men are more likely to eat excessively in response to feeling stressed or upset, whereas women are more likely to eat excessively in response to failing a diet in certain communities.

The symptoms of a rise in the hormone cortisol, which is one of the body's reactions to stress, are believed to be close to those of the drug prednisone. Both appear to trigger the body's stress mechanism (fight or flight), which includes elevated pulse and respiratory rates, the blood supply to tissues, and visual acuity. Increased appetite is also a part of the stress reaction to provide the body with the strength it requires to combat or escape, resulting in cravings for so-called comfort foods. People that have been exposed to persistent stress (such as work, education, or family stress, or exposure to violence or abuse) are more likely to have excessively elevated cortisol levels in their bodies, which may lead to the development of chronic emotional-eating habits.

Emotional eating is a psychological condition in which people associate food with warmth, strength, good emotions, or some other cause other than supplying nutrition to their bodies. When they are physically complete, they can eat to fill an emotional void and indulge in mindless eating. Some people who eat their emotions may have been raised to associate food with feelings rather than sustenance, particularly if the food was limited or often used as a reward or punishment, or as a replacement for emotional intimacy.

What are the signs and symptoms of emotional eating?

A desire to become painfully hungry all of a time, rather than steadily as in a real physical urge to eat triggered by an empty stomach, is one of the warning signs of emotional eating. Emotional eaters are more likely to consume fast food than to seek out healthy meals, and the need to eat is normally accompanied by tension or an unpleasant feeling, such as depression, disappointment, rage, remorse, or annoyance. Other characteristics of emotional eating include a loss of control when eating and frequent regret over what has been consumed.

What types of Professionals deal with emotional eating?

When emotional eating leads to overweight or obesity, a variety of health care providers may assess and manage it, as well as assist in weight loss. Since this symptom can appear at any point during a person's existence, it can be addressed by anyone from pediatricians to family doctors to other primary care physicians. Emotional-eating patients can be cared for by clinicians, medical practitioners, and physician assistants. Psychiatrists, behavioral psychologists, social workers, and certified counselors are among the mental health providers who are often interested in identifying and addressing this issue. Although all of these professionals can assist patients who suffer from emotional eating, it's possible that more than one of them will collaborate to help the individual solve this symptom.

What approaches do physicians use to recognize emotional eating?

After confirming that the sufferer has undergone a clinical assessment and test work to ensure that the disorder is not part of a neurological or other medical illness like Prader-Willi syndrome, the diagnosis of emotional eating is created. The patient might be asked a set of questions from a structured questionnaire or self-test as part of the behavioral wellbeing portion of the assessment to better determine the presence of emotional eating. Emotional eating can be differentiated from such eating conditions such as bulimia, binge eating, or pica by a thorough examination of the background of mental health symptoms. A mental well-being specialist will likely look to see whether there are any other mental disorders involved.

Notes:

Chapter: 2. Myths That are True

Comfort foods are distinct for men and women

There is a differentiation between men and women. Men prefer soft, hearty, meal-related comfort foods (think roast, casseroles, and soup), while women prefer snack foods, according to research (think chocolate and ice cream).

Feeling guilty for eating cake has a negative impact on weight reduction

Eating cake while feeling guilty leads to a slower weight loss. The cake is comfort food that is often linked to feelings of regret and worry, as well as satisfaction and relaxation. Dieters who correlated cake with "guilt" rather than "celebration" were less likely to lose weight in one report. Dieters who experienced happy emotions, such as joy and warmth from the cake, were more likely to lose weight. Guilt has the power to derail your efforts.

We crave familiar comfort foods

We consume comfort foods because it's what we've always done. When we're nervous, we return to the things we consume most, whether they're safe or not. Students were more inclined to select the snacks they consume more often at high tension periods, according to researchers who followed their eating patterns among college students during midterm exams. Choosing common foods needs less thinking and commitment.

Ritual provides a sense of security

Ritual provides a sense of security and pleasure. Will you have a favorite way to consume comfort foods? Do you really take the icing off the cupcake first, or do you always split the peanut butter sandwich in half? Food is consumed in a variety of forms by most of us. And the positive emotions we get from these little routines are backed up by science. Eaters who created a custom out of unwrapping and progressively splitting bits of a chocolate bar not only felt the pleasant relaxation emotions, but they also liked the chocolate better than those who just unwrapped and consumed the chocolate, according to a report reported in the journal Psychological Research.

Eating is an act of emotion

It's not all about the flavor. We also assume that comfort foods taste good whether they taste good or that consuming them feels good. In a study published in the Journal of Clinical Investigation, researchers were able to evoke the same emotions and memories by inserting a fat-based substance directly into the stomachs of the subjects. The researchers then caused depression in the participants and discovered that those who obtained the fat-based solution had a lower brain reaction to sadness on MRI tests than those who received the dummy or placebo solution. Many that were given the "comfort" cure didn't have that much pain. This prompted the researchers to believe that something hormonal is activated in the gut, and then sends messages to the brain, making us feel healthy.

Happy people overeat too

Emotional eating is triggered by both positive and negative emotions. According to the journal, sometimes positive thoughts cause cravings for comfort foods. In reality, positive people are more prone to overeat than sad people, which is a little-known fact.

Chicken soup is a perfect company

Chicken soup is soothing and will help you feel less lonely. This is why: People who consumed chicken noodle soup were less sad when consuming it, according to a report reported in Psychological Research. They were also able to come up with more relational terms to explain their emotions while eating it. To put it another way, if you consume the soup when chatting to others, you're more likely to speak with them. Comfort meals equal soothing emotions, which equals comfort in the company of others.

We always need comfort food

At the end of the day, comfort is sought. Take a peek at some of the more popular "last meals" requested by death row inmates: Fried foods were chosen by 67 percent, and desserts by 66 percent. Is it so surprising that they crave calorie-dense comfort foods?

While you're away from family, familiar foods are comforting

Eating common comfort foods, according to a survey of students studying abroad in England, offered emotional help and provided a "taste of home" comfort. If you live abroad for a long time, experts warn that you'll start to miss the fresh foods in your acculturated diet in the same way you craved your native land's comfort foods.

Dieters are the ones that are more vulnerable to comfort food

Dieters are the people that are more likely to feed mentally. People who are at risk for emotional eating under stress, according to experts, have a high BMI, express "low" or "moody" emotions, and have a high cortisol reactivity (your body's response to stress). However, studies have shown that attempting to step back and exercise discipline usually backfires!

The level of comfort is dose-dependent

That's right! When emotional eaters were offered a small amount of chocolate (about one-ninth of a Hershey's bar), there were no shifts of attitude. Unfortunately, it took a lot of chocolate to even create a dent in attitude, and as we have learned, it's just a temporary "feel nice" practice!

Chapter 3. Myths that are False

Myth #1: Emotional eating is not the same as all types of eating

Eating is an intense experience. Attempts to exclude emotion from eating improve the implicit motivation to consume foods with higher emotional and sensory quality (taste, smell, texture, sweet, salty, fat). That's why broccoli is never a good substitute for chocolate.

Attempts to eliminate emotion from eating lead to "deprivation motivations," an urge to get as many as possible because supplies last when availability is restricted or prohibited. Note that only one tiny slice of fruit was prohibited to Adam and Eve; equate that to the list of items we're not supposed to consume on diets.

Since we can't take the emotion out of food, long-term weight loss is based on which emotions drive us. The choice is to choose between core pain and core worth.

Disregard, insignificance, shame, devaluation, disrespect, rejection, powerlessness, inadequacy, or unlovability are all feeling the core hurt eating seeks to stop. It's impossible to ignore the connection between core pain and high-energy, high-sensory food. For a few minutes, fast eating of high sensory, high-calorie food numbs pain and restores vitality; for a few minutes, rapid eating of high sensory, high-calorie food numbs pain and restores energy.

Quick eating causes core pain. We realize that if we stop, our core pains will worsen and our vitality will disappear. As a result, we don't rest unless our bodies tell us to. Overeating becomes "attacks on food" when central hurts are serious and the ability to control them is underdeveloped, rendering food harmful rather than nourishing, an instrument of damage rather than a source of well-being and well-being.

Eating is a type of self-expression. Rather than dwelling on what you don't have, you reflect on increasing the meaning of your life. It encourages you to move your attention away from weight and diet and toward love toward yourself and others. When you place a higher priority on yourself, you will naturally place a higher value on your fitness and well-being, and you will learn to inspire yourself by "acts of kindness."

Myth #2: If I lose weight, I would have a higher self-esteem

Weight loss plans emphasize this message both clearly and implicitly by emphasizing "goals" and "orders," as in "Think of how you don't like looking in the mirror."

"You should embrace yourself overweight," they might suggest, or "Keep walking, even though you relapse." Yet no amount of lip service will substitute for the mental effects of goals: if you don't meet them, you're a loser.

Over-eaters already sound like failures when it comes to weight management. But, just in case it wasn't enough to guarantee defeat, weight reduction plans' targets and rules have a built-in failure mechanism, simply because all winners are also losers. We sacrifice as much as we gain in something that lasts a long period, such as a lifelong motivation to feed. It's just regression to the mean; once you collect enough data, such as test scores, the mean result, or average score, becomes more common when anomalies from the mean become less so.

If you "gain" by hitting your weight reduction target, figures suggest that you would most definitely "lose" by relapsing at some stage in your life (hopefully earlier rather than later). "I dropped 200 pounds this year, but I added 210," goes the old joke. Goals and guidelines around food are more apt to elicit core hurts (guilty and insufficient) than core values, setting you up for failure.

The weakest aspect of this misconception — that you would love yourself more if you lose weight — is that it distorts a plain truth: You will not lose weight until you value yourself more.

Is it the loved self or the devalued self that is more prone to binge eat and attack food (or to be a bad partner or abuser, for that matter)?

Myth #3: We eat so much when we're bored

Boredom's innate motivation is to pursue something interesting to do. You don't eat to escape boredom; instead, you get involved in something. Boredom just encourages people to overeat as it threatens their heart hurts. When boredom makes me feel unimportant or insufficient, my subconscious misinterprets the decline in energy and well-being as hunger, raising my odds of overeating.

Myth #4: We eat to feel better

Many publications have encouraged us to create lists of our "favorite foods," which include items like pizza, oatmeal, cookies, chicken and dumplings, ice cream, and so on. The manufacturers of alcohol and Valium would be out of business if these foods provided substantial comforting qualities.

It has little to do with the food and more to do with their core principle, why certain people feel comforted after consuming those foods. They get the impression that they are "taking care of themselves," because they should not overeat. When a central principle motivates food (or something else), relaxation and overall well-being are possible outcomes.

However, if core hurts drive "comfort food," the outcome would be remorse and shame. When you think about it, it's a little silly to suggest you consume for pleasure when overeating creates serious physical and emotional pain.

Myth #5: We eat because we enjoy it (because our mothers expressed affection with food).

This is a particularly harmful myth. Over-eaters of missing mothers are advised that they eat for attention because their mothers did not show devotion for food from the very individuals who support it. Ok, guess what? Food is a fairly popular way to show love. In general, most mothers use food to show love to their children, even those who grow up to be thin; nevertheless, parents who make a huge deal of the type of food their children consume are more likely to have eating disorders.

Aside from empirical evidence, "eating for love," like "eating for warmth," defies logic. Overeating contributes to self-loathing and resentment, but not to affection. Is anybody ever experienced love as a result of overeating? If we did, we'd savor it, prolong it, and stretch it out as far as possible. Overeaters, particularly those who attack food, have a tendency to eat at a single speed: quick and furious. Some people will binge until they are completely satisfied, only to feel so terrible for themselves that they will finally adhere to their weight reduction targets. Self-loathing, on the other hand, just encourages you to engage in self-destructive acts.

Since core hurt eating is not an effort to feel appreciated, welcomed, or cherished, we don't eat for affection. Core wounds, on the other hand, are about feeling incapable of worth, recognition, and affection. A feeling of unworthiness triggers a significant drop in well-being and energy, which strengthens the need to feed.

Eating is a pleasurable experience

True, but it's just for three minutes. Research published in the Journal of Appetite looked into how long chocolate makes you feel healthy. Comfort and bliss, it turned out, just last 3 minutes. Three minutes! Isn't it amazing how brief comfort food can be?

Everybody suffers from the same hunger pangs

Comfort items aren't universal. Do you think chocolate is the world's favorite feel-good food? It's not the case. People in various countries seek relief from various foods. Miso soup, okay (rice porridge served to sick children), and ramen are common comfort foods in Japan. Samosas, potato-stuffed crisps served with spicy green chutney, are a common snack in India. It's new pasta or potato gnocchi in Italy.

Hormones are responsible for chocolate cravings

Hormonal chocolate cravings are not triggered by PMS. You may believe that the hormones cause you to desire chocolate at the time of the month, but despite no longer getting periods, 80 percent of menopausal women experience chocolate cravings. Experts agree that our need for warmth, coupled with our anxiety regarding our cycle, drives us to use a culturally reinforced coping mechanism. To put it another way, we expect chocolate to benefit, so we continue to desire it, rather than hormones leading us to it.

When it comes to comfort meals, money is irrelevant

Among those on public assistance, Kraft macaroni isn't much of a comfort. The famous Kraft macaroni and cheese dinner is often listed as a comfort meal among middle-income people who do not struggle to pay for food. For some who aren't sure how they'll budget for their next meal, though, it's just the same. Since this cheesy packaged lunch is often given to food banks, it runs the risk of being a monotonous staple for recipients, reinforcing their loss of financial strength and meal options.

Chapter 4. Solutions of Emotional Eating

4.1. Useful Suggestions

1. A few useful suggestions should be implemented while we are feeling both up and down in times of celebration, joy, or down while we might be feeling down or nervous in an attempt to disrupt this loop of possible addiction or emotional intake of food, and they include the following.

2. Maintaining a food diary about what you consume, how much you eat, how hungry you are, and how you feel during the day will help you find causes.

3. Reducing discomfort that could be leading to overeating or reward eating by going on a stroll, breathing exercises, yoga, or engaging in a favorite hobby.

4. Do a hunger fact check to determine if you are experiencing physical or mental hunger.

5. Seek assistance from relatives, friends, or treatment staff.

6. Combat boredom by contacting a mate, heading for a stroll, playing a game, listening to music, or reading to prevent the mind from drifting to food-related thinking.

7. Remove the lure by making your home and office a secure refuge free of things that are commonly borrowed for convenience.

8. Don't deny yourself of anything. We cannot deny ourselves fundamental needs like food, unlike those recovering from opioid abuse or alcoholism who would abstain from such drugs. Cravings may be exacerbated by putting too many restrictions on yourself or eating the same ingredients over and over. To bring diversity to your diet, consume a satisfying amount of nutritious foods and indulge in a treat every now and then.

9. Snack on fruits, vegetables, nuts, and un-buttered popcorn for a nutritious snack.

10. Learn from your mistakes: Whenever you have an emotional eating crisis, forgive yourself and try again with your next meal. Do not write off the day or yourself as a total disappointment. We are just human, and life happens. We will always fall into these traps, and how we survive and evolve will determine our success. Learn from the experience and make constructive changes to avoid such occurrences in the future.

4.2. What is the right way to cope with emotional eating?

Overcoming emotional eating typically involves educating the sufferer healthy ways to perceive food and cultivate improved eating behaviors, as well as identifying their reasons for participating in this behavior and improving effective stress prevention and coping strategies.

1. Exercise is an effective part of stress management since it reduces the release of stress hormones, which may contribute to a reduction of depression, anxiety, and insomnia, as well as a decline in the propensity to partake in emotional eating.

2. Meditation and other calming strategies are both efficient methods to relieve depression and, as a result, minimize emotional eating. As a consequence, performing one to two mediation exercises per day may have long-term health advantages, including reducing elevated blood pressure and heart rate.

3. Other effective strategies to effectively alleviate stress include abstaining from opioid usage and drinking no more than small levels of alcohol since both of these drugs heighten the body's reaction to stress. Indulging in the usage of such drugs often prohibits the individual from confronting their issues head-on, preventing them from developing successful coping or stress-reduction strategies.

4. Such stress-reducing lifestyle improvements include having breaks at home and at college. Avoid cramming so much into your schedule. Recognize the stressors and react appropriately. Take daily vacation days at times that are comfortable for you. Structure your life so that you can adapt to the unpredictable in a relaxed manner.

5. Psychotropic drugs, especially selective serotonin reuptake inhibitors (SSRIs), may be incredibly effective if stress triggers a full-blown psychological condition such as posttraumatic stress disorder (PTSD), clinical depression, or anxiety disorders. Sertraline (Zoloft), paroxetine (Paxil), fluoxetine (Prozac), citalopram (Celexa), and escitalopram are examples of SSRIs (Lexapro).

4.3. What are the chances of emotional eating if left untreated?

Emotional overeating, if left unchecked, will contribute to problems such as difficulty losing weight, obesity, and even the initiation of food addiction. People who are vulnerable to emotional eating, on the other hand, are also more open to stress mitigation in correcting their propensity to emotionally eat than people who eat less while stressed.

4.4.   Is there a way to avoid emotional eating?

Reduced discomfort, healthy approaches to consider and control feelings, and treating food as sustenance rather than a means to fix issues are also essential factors in avoiding emotional eating (eating to live rather than living to eat). Emotional eating is often prevented by dreaming about the potential rather than focusing on meeting food cravings, according to research. Meditation, yoga, and other positive tension prevention and stress management strategies, as well as limiting caffeine, alcohol, and medications, are also good approaches to avoid unhealthy eating habits.

Conclusion

The blunt truth to this issue is that it does happen, and it is not restricted to women. It is important to have a safe or positive relationship with food. Many of what we do as a group revolves around the idea of using food to commemorate both happy and sad events of our lives. Comfort foods like fried chicken, burgers, and casseroles are high in fat; high sweet products like sweets, desserts, and pies are high in sugar; and high starch items like bread, rice, and pasta are high in carbohydrate. We seldom pause to consider how these events would affect us at the moment. Its aim is to fill a hole. Our ingestion of these foods will trigger our brain's instant reward receptors, making us feel happier and need more. A person or community stress-management treatment may be really beneficial for those who require assistance coping with stress. Stress counseling and community therapy have been found to enhance mental well-being and reduce stress symptoms.

This insatiable need or drive is similar to an addiction, and it exists regardless of our appetite. These habits can lead to an unbalanced diet, which can accelerate the development of obesity. The bidirectional relationship between our mood and obesity becomes entangled, allowing each disease state to feed off the other. It's likely that you'll feel sad or nervous as a consequence of your weight. The framework of "When I'm down, I eat to feel stronger" on the other side, may become a constant feedback loop and cycle that causes an individual to suffer. This book will provide you a real insight into the Myths and Realities of

Emotional Eating and comprehensive coping-strategies to fight your fears and to become emotionally independent well-being.

Notes: